Are Common Heart Skip Palpitations Dangerous?

Premature Ventricular and Atrial Contractions (PVCs and PACs)

By: James M. Lowrance © 2012

Dedication:

To the many people who suffer from benign but often anxiety-producing skipped heartbeat palpitations. May you find comfort from the information contained within the chapters of this book -- written by someone who has experienced these palpitations at many points in my life for over 30 years.

-Jim Lowrance

TABLE OF CONTENTS:

Are Common Heart Skip Palpitations Dangerous?

INTRODUCTION:

Skipped heartbeats occur in most, if not 100% of the general population, at some point during their lives. Some medical sources state that about half of us experience them on a relatively frequent basis. For some people however, these heart palpitations called "Premature Ventricular Contractions" and "Premature Atrial Contractions" (PVCs and PACs), occur at a frequency or forcefulness, that can be concerning to them and that can result in chronic anxiety and/or panic attacks. In most cases these palpitations are benign but the unpleasant feeling they may cause can at times override any reassurance one might receive by a doctor, that their heart is otherwise healthy and normal.

It would seem that some individuals are more aware of their skipped heartbeats than are others, which in-reality are extra heartbeats (extra systole: ectopic heartbeats) that cause the sensation of missed ones. Many people with PVCs and/or PACs, are finely tuned-in to the symptoms these may cause and once anxiety over them is added, they can occur with more force and frequency.

Are Common Heart Skip Palpitations Dangerous?

In most cases anxiety and stress precedes and triggers them. While this still does not make them dangerous, according to many reputable heart specialists, the fear and anticipation of them can degrade a person's quality of life. It in-essence becomes an anxiety disorder in itself or is added to an existing one, causing a worsening of symptoms.

It is my intention, through the chapters of this book, to inform readers who experience these common but most-often benign palpitations, with facts, that can help them to better-cope with the concerning symptoms they may experience with these strange heartbeats.

CHAPTER ONE

Understanding Premature Ventricular and Atrial Contractions

Just Exactly What are these Heart Skip Palpitations?

Premature Ventricular Contractions (PVCs - originating from the lower heart valves) and Premature Atrial Contractions (PACs - originating from the upper heart valves) are mild and usually benign cardiac events, that can cause some degree of symptoms but that are usually not life restricting, other than the possible mental stress and anxiety that can accompany them. While people who experience these disrhythmias are usually at no risk for any type of negative consequence from experiencing them, many will find it very hard not to be concerned about them, even after reassurance by their medical doctors, who inform them that the palpitations (unusual sensations from the heart), are harmless.

I cannot fault those individuals who do experience anxiety resulting from PVCs and/or PACS.

Are Common Heart Skip Palpitations Dangerous?

I personally began to experience these skipping heartbeats, in my teen years and the very unusual feeling they produced, which can be described as a pause in heartbeats, followed by a thump-sensation in the chest. Mine have continued to occur intermittently and I am now one birthday away from being 50 years old at the time of this writing. So far, I have seen no ill effect from them, other than the panic and anxiety symptoms I have experienced with them on occasion. Now, when I begin to see them manifest, I can usually ignore them, since gaining the knowledge that they are harmless in the vast majority of cases, although I will admit that when they occur with frequency or in multiples, I can still find myself feeling anxious.

I actually made an office visit with a cardiologist in the year 2001, after experiencing a long period of frequent PVCs/PACs and my results from a stress electrocardiogram, showed no abnormalities in my heart rhythm or any suspected blockage in any of my heart vessels or valves. Another reason I scheduled the visit with a heart specialist, was due to my being diagnosed with a heart murmur, in my teens.

A medical doctor, who was treating me at the time for a condition unrelated to my heart, heard the murmur during my visit with him, at about age 15. He informed my parents and recommended that we schedule an appointment with a cardiologist. Upon being examined and having heart testing conducted, including an EKG, a heart ex-ray and cardiac ultrasound (echocardiogram), the cardiologist concluded that I was experiencing "Wolff-Parkinson-White Syndrome" (WPWS); a potentially serious heart murmur. He explained to both my parents and me, that this meant that I basically had an extra electrical pathway in my heart, that was causing a faster rhythm or what is also referred to as "tachycardia". He also informed us that he felt the murmur was of a mild variety in the category of the heart murmur.

The cardiologist I saw in 2001, stated that the previous diagnosis was incorrect because the murmur was not found during the more recent testing and that the previous heart specialist was mistaken. He informed me that he specializes in cases of WPWS and that he had published studies he was involved with, in researching the murmur.

He also stated that if I actually had the condition, it would still be present and unchanged without surgical correction of it. While I was relieved to receive the all-clear more than 20 years later, I now realize that the diagnosis I was given in my teens, caused me to become more "heartbeat conscious". My fear of the heart murmur, was causing me to monitor my cardiac activity much closer and I found myself taking my pulse frequently and paying close attention to the speed of my heart rhythm. I had actually begun to experience infrequent episodes of panic sensations even previous to my knowledge of having the heart murmur, which I apparently outgrew or that was misdiagnosed. I also began to have ongoing problems with free-floating anxiety as well (generalized feelings of anxiousness), which became chronic as years passed and that eventually fit the definition of "generalized Anxiety Disorder", by the time I reached 19 years of age.

This is also the approximate time I began experiencing the heart-skip palpitations, which genuinely caused me to fear what was occurring within my heart.

Are Common Heart Skip Palpitations Dangerous?

I attributed these to the heart murmur and I believed this to be the case for nearly two decades before receiving the counter-diagnoses at age 38. My episodes of the skipping heartbeats, would occur following long episodes of stress or anxiety or after I had consumed too many stimulants in my diet (i.e. caffeine, alcohol or refined sugars). I noticed that I would experience them for days, weeks or even for months at a time, with periods of relief from them in-between, that were months or even years in duration. I now believe that these symptoms I was experiencing, including the tachycardia as a teen, were actually caused by a condition known as "Mitral Valve Prolapse" (MVP), which is a common murmur found in the general population and that can become a "syndrome" (MVPS), when symptoms are caused by it.

In addition to heart skip palpitations and other heart rhythm changes, MVP-Syndrome, can also result in the symptoms of dizziness, sensitivities to stimulants, fatigue, blood pressure changes (usually low -- hypotension) and shortness of breath.

Are Common Heart Skip Palpitations Dangerous?

I also believe MVP to be the heart murmur that was originally detected in me, due to both of my parents having been diagnosed with it in their 70s and my daughter being diagnosed with a benign heart murmur in her pre-teens (it is highly hereditary). MVP itself, which is also referred to as a "click murmur" (describing the sound it sometimes produces when monitored by stethoscope), is also a usually-benign condition but that is notorious for causing heart skip palpitations (more on MVP/MVPS later).

I feel that my previous diagnoses of WPWS, began a vicious cycle of increased anxiety for me, which led to my experiences with PVCs/PACs. The sensation of a pause in the heartbeat caused by these disrhythmias is actually caused by "extra heartbeats", also referred to as "ectopic" and "extrasystole" heartbeats. These can be fairly rare in occurrence for many people or they may occur with relative frequency however, even the latter is not usually of concern in the vast majority of cases. Some individuals may also experience them, with every other heartbeat (bigeminy) or every third heartbeat (trigeminy) or every fourth heartbeat (quadrigeminy).

Are Common Heart Skip Palpitations Dangerous?

They may also be more erratic, so that different variations of normal beats, followed by the disrhythmic beats are occurring.

Some people may experience several PVCs/PACs in a row (i.e. couplets = 2, triplets = 3, etc...) but even experiencing multiples is not of concern, unless a run of them remains sustained/constant for more than 30 seconds at a time, with no normal heartbeats in-between, which would then fall under the category of "tachycardia". In most cases, runs of skip heartbeat palpitations, fall under the category of "Non-Sustained Ventricular Tachycardia" (NSVT) and even this is usually considered a harmless event if the non-sustained periods are not frequent or occurring for more than 30 seconds at a time.

While statistics vary, some medical sources believe that half of us experience these sometimes irritating palpitations (likely closer to 100%) and that only about 30% actually notice them. Most doctors will not give them much credence, unless a patient also complains that the ectopic heartbeats are accompanied by significant lightheadedness, fainting, shortness of breath or chest pain.

Are Common Heart Skip Palpitations Dangerous?

If a patient complains about one of these co-morbid symptoms, a doctor might recommend cardiac testing or a visit to a heart specialist. In many cases, the symptoms are not directly related to the palpitations but may be a manifestation of co-occurring anxiety or from an unrelated health disorder (i.e. acid reflux, asthma or joint/muscle pain). Even without significant co-morbid symptoms, some patients will need to see a cardiologist, in order to experience peace-of-mind, knowing that they have good heart-health and that the palpitations will not lead to any serious event. The disrhythmias can be of slightly-higher concern when experienced by the elderly, by those with hypertensive conditions (high blood pressure) or by those who have known heart problems but they otherwise pose no dangers to those who experience them, who are relatively heart-healthy.

I recently received a comment from a lady who read one of my resources that contained information on the PVC/PAC subject and she complained about my not offering more substantial information regarding how to get rid of them. I responded to her comment with the reply that follows below.

Are Common Heart Skip Palpitations Dangerous?

My Reply:

"I felt it might add perspective to mention that there has so far not been a treatment developed that rids sufferers of PVCs, of their heart-skip palpitations (some patients are referred for "ablations"- destruction of small area of heart tissue but most doctors feel this is too-risky for benign heart palpitations -- same is true of drugs that are specifically-designed to control abnormal heart beats).

Certainly some people with the condition have found relief from certain things such as supplementing with omega-3 essential oils (fish oil caplets) potassium or magnesium; to relieve or completely resolve their PVCs but others trying these very same supplements and see little or see no improvement.

With this being the case, every book or info source you find on the subject, will contain basically the same information regarding lifestyle changes to improve PVCs, such as stress-reduction, exercise, beta-blockers, anti-anxiety drugs and avoiding stimulants in the diet.

Are Common Heart Skip Palpitations Dangerous?

Giving heart-skip palpitation sufferers reassurance that PVCs will not harm someone with a structurally normal heart is in my opinion, possibly the most effective method in helping them to cope with them and in some cases, this actually helps them to overcome them completely (in many cases this requires the aid of a psychologist). The reason being that fear of PVCs actually triggers them because they can be fueled and literally caused by adrenaline surges, such as those experienced by anxiety disorder sufferers. I -in-fact believe a PVC Syndrome should be included in the list of known, major anxiety disorders. While I do give the same type info found via online sources on the PVC subject in my articles and books/eBooks, I concentrate a great deal of the information on helping PVCers not fear the symptoms of these devilish little heart palpitations.

When it comes to health conditions and diseases, I personally have yet to find a book/eBook with information that is not already found online. I also believe with firm conviction that this can serve as frustration to those who order a new health title and find that it repeats basically the same information they have previously found online.

Are Common Heart Skip Palpitations Dangerous?

This is specially true of those with difficulty coping or who have severe cases of a particular health problem.

At the same time, there are those who are new to a health condition or who prefer not to conduct lengthy online search to connect the major info-aspects of a health disorder all together for a better perspective on them. If one is lucky, they find free online sources that do cover all major aspects of a subject but this is not usually the case and successful online search requires putting-in exactly-correct combinations of search terms, otherwise certain sets of information remain obscure. Sometimes, even the most obvious search-terms do not yield the specific information they are seeking (I have experienced this problem myself on many occasions).

There simply is no "magic bullet" for curing PVCs and I for one would love to see one be developed because I am a patient who suffers with these and at times mine can be very frequent and sometimes concerning. The reassurance that they do not cause heart damage in those with otherwise normal hearts, has been a major help in coping for me personally." **End of Reply**

CHAPTER TWO

Heart-Skip Palpitations (PVCs) and Cardiomyopathy

(Heart Enlargement Risk with Premature Ventricular Contractions?)

As noted earlier, according to reputable heart doctors about half (50%) of the population experiences PVC – heart-skip palpitations. Some people have them far more frequently than others due to factors such as anxiety/stress and use of stimulants.

The cardiomyopathy scare that some people with frequent PVCs have after online search can be easily remedied by asking their doctors for a simple BNP blood test (B-Type Naturietic Peptide). This test detects both restrictive and constrictive cardiomyopathy, which always presents with degrees of heart enlargement and has 98% accuracy, according to The Harvard Medical School. Cardiomyopathy is also called Chronic Heart Failure and Congestive Heart Failure and even mild cases of it can be detected via the BNP blood test, which is also not expensive to have done.

Are Common Heart Skip Palpitations Dangerous?

Of course an echocardiogram is an even more detailed test for looking at the heart but not everyone has health insurance or can afford to see a cardiologist to have one performed.

BNP Normal Values

The BNP levels they look for in people with mild heart failure is "100" and above in a range of 0 to 100. This would indicate mild cardiomyopathy. If the result comes in at 300 to 600, this indicates moderate heart failure and results at above 600, indicate severe heart failure. I would strongly suspect that the 2% loss of accuracy out of 98% involves those readings that are close to borderline because the higher readings are certain for heart enlargement.

BNP is actually a hormone released from the brain, in response to added pressure of any kind on the heart muscle and it will elevate even if there is stress on only one heart valve, such as the left ventricle or even if a person has chronic (long-term) untreated, severe hypertension that has placed added stress and pressure on the heart. If chronic PVCs have done this same thing (likely extremely rare, unless other heart disease is also present), the BNP will elevate.

Are Common Heart Skip Palpitations Dangerous?

My BNP Test Results

I had the BNP test ordered by my doctor, one year ago, after I developed adult asthma, that I felt certain was due to my chronic GERD (acid reflux), which I have had most of my life. With the fact however that heart enlargement can also cause breathing problems (cardiac asthma), I had the test ordered, plus a chest ex-ray, which showed normal size heart. My BNP result came back at "4", which I was very happy with.

A few weeks ago, I had the BNP repeated after the onset of my most recent phase of PVCs and my result was very low again, at "16" -- still far below the "100" upper-normal cut-off value. This despite weeks of increase in my daily walking routine (doubled my distance) and the fact that the blood was drawn in the afternoon, rather than in the morning as the previous one was. BNP, like other hormones, will fluctuate several points within a 24 hour period and it also increases naturally with age. I'm close to the half-century mark age-wise myself, so I'm very happy with my two low readings over the one-year period I had them done.

Are Common Heart Skip Palpitations Dangerous?

Heart Failure Risk in PVC Sufferers with otherwise Normal Hearts

For those who may have had a bit of cyberchondria rise up in their anxiety-sensitive hearts regarding heart failure, resulting from online search regarding PVCs, I wanted to add this bit of information for balance. Also keep in mind that literally 100s of online posts have been published by PVC sufferers, who have them very frequently, for decades and they still report having healthy heart check-ups. Those who do develop heart disease following years of PVCs, could have a number of other factors involved (i.e. smoking, morbid obesity, severe untreated hypertension, heart defects or they are elderly etc...) and the PVCs may have had little or no involvement in the development of their cardiac diseases.

When heart disease is actually present, PVCs can be of some concern (some doctors state only slightly higher risks), as can many other things that are of far-less concern in people with otherwise health hearts.

The Real Scoop Regarding Congestive Heart Failure (Cardiomyopathy)

I will now add information regarding Congestive Heart Failure, for those readers who would like to know what this illness is really all-about and how it manifests.

Congestive Heart Failure (CHF) is more common in people ages 65 and older but can affect people at any age who have defects or damage to their heart muscles. In most patients, CHF has a chronic course but can be reversed in some cases. Even when it remains chronic (ongoing) treatments can be administered to treat symptoms and to improve quality of life for CHF patients. In some cases, fluid may build in a patient's lungs and/or their heart may become enlarged but there are treatments to relieve symptoms caused by complications of CHF.

Symptoms of CHF

The symptoms can vary among individuals, but the ones that are typically experienced may include the following:

* Shortness of breath
* Wheezing and coughing ...

Are Common Heart Skip Palpitations Dangerous?

* Edema in the ankles and/or abdomen (swelling)
* Fatigue
* Heart enlargement
* Exercise intolerance
* Failure in other organs of the body (i.e. the kidneys, liver and brain)

These symptoms occur due to a weakening of the heart muscle over time, which causes inadequate supply of blood circulation to the muscles and organs of the body. A resulting effect of diminished heart function out-put, includes a build-up of fluid around the heart and in the lungs, which also contributes to symptoms.

Causes of CHF

Conditions that cause serious heart arrhythmias (rather than the benign types) and damage to the heart muscle can result in the development of CHF over time. If a person has a severe heart murmur or a birth defect in the heart, for example (congenital heart defect) this can cause the condition to develop as they age and especially when they reach their senior-age years.

Heart attacks can also contribute to the development of CHF due to the resulting damage in the heart muscle that causes less-adequate heart function as a person ages. As the heart muscle struggles to supply proper blood circulation output while it is in a damaged or inadequately functioning state, it will often become enlarged. This is its attempt to allow more blood-flow through the heart valves but is a serious development that can require emergency care.

Lifestyle Treatments for CHF

If the condition is mild to moderate and not causing significant symptoms, a treating doctor might simply prescribe lifestyle changes and intermittent short-term use of a diuretic medication (for fluid retention).

These changes in lifestyle might include the following:

* Losing excess weight in the body

* Regular exercise at proper tolerance level

* A healthy diet

* Reduced fluid intake ...

Are Common Heart Skip Palpitations Dangerous?

...

* Removing sodium from the diet (salt – which results in fluid retention)

This type of regimen would be monitored closely by regular follow ups with the patient, to see if the treatment is working or if prescription medications need to be added.

Prescription and Surgical Treatments

Prescribed medications for more severe cases might include beta-blocker drugs to control hypertension, cardiac glycosides to increase cardiac output and ACE Inhibitors to prevent renin released by the kidneys from converting into angiotensin II (a hormone that causes heart constriction).

Should CHF worsen despite prescribed treatments, these worst-case scenarios might require corrective surgery for damaged or malfunctioning heart valves or for stints to be implanted to open constricted arteries. Rarely, a patient will be recommended for heart transplant if they are determined to be an approved candidate for one.

Are Common Heart Skip Palpitations Dangerous?

This would mean they are otherwise healthy, so that their body will not reject the replaced organ.

In many cases, the prognosis for CHF can be good with proper treatment and with close monitoring of treated patients by a qualified MD or cardiologist.

CHAPTER THREE

Do PVCs and PACs Increase the Risk for Premature Death?

(The Fear caused by Frequent Skips and Thumps)

I would hope to provide further comfort to those who experience these common heart palpitations, with frequency but I would also recommend that a medical doctor be consulted for further reassurance, when one is experiencing an irregular heartbeat of any type. While most heart palpitations are benign (harmless) some can indicate a structural problem within the heart muscle that requires treatment.

Skips and Thumps

PVCs and PACs are often felt by the one experiencing them, as a pause in the heartbeat, followed by a thump sensation in the chest, neck or abdomen and they are very common as previously mentioned. Due to the fact that they are experienced by such a large portion of the general population, huge numbers of posts regarding them can be found on heart-health medical forums online.

Are Common Heart Skip Palpitations Dangerous?

In some cases, patients are warning their fellow-patients, about the risk these palpitations have for causing eventual heart failure or sudden death from cardiac arrest. This type of information does however need to be seasoned with some perspective, based on reliable medical information, so as not to be ambiguous regarding realistic risk factors.

Many PVC/PAC Patients Report Good Heart Health

According to the information I found on reputable medical sources, regarding these common heart palpitations, heart disease **is not** the most common cause of PVCs/PACs. If that were the case, the estimated 50% of the general population, estimated to have relatively frequent PVCs/PACs, would all be walking around with heart disease.

I have seen literally 1,000s of posts by frequent PVC/PAC sufferers, whose cardiologists ruled out structural heart disease of any kind via complete workups (i.e. stress test/EKG and echocardiograms) and yet they experience these horrible-feeling pause-thumps, on a daily bases.

28

Many relate having experienced them since their childhood and yet they were still given a clean bill of heart health in their 30s, 40s or 50s, by their cardiologists.

More on Palpitations and Cardiomyopathy

In regard to cardiomyopathy, which was discussed in a previous chapter (weakening of the heart muscle), PVCs/PACs should not place any more stress on the heart than would normal activities that increase the heart rate (i.e. exercise, excitement and sex), because the premature beat that happens with PVCs/PACs, is simply that...a double-beat. This would be equal to two heartbeats that simply occur closer together.

People who do develop cardiomyopathy with years of constant PVCs/PACs, likely had a propensity or predisposition toward developing it and the palpitations were simply a contributing factor. I will add that in rare cases, it's possibly a direct cause of heart failure but likely far more of a possibility in senior age people and/or in those who already have serious co-morbid health problems. I base this on my search/research on many medical websites that specialize in heart health information.

Are Common Heart Skip Palpitations Dangerous?

I recently viewed a YouTube video by Dr. Stephen Sinatra, a Board Certified Cardiologist, in which he states these facts, plus admits the he also experiences PVCs, as did many of his fellow students, which they discovered when they were studying for their medical credentials. He mentions "stress" in the video, as a precipitating factor for the occurrence of these palpitations, in students pursuing their educational degrees to practice professional medicine.

The Diagnostic Value of Common Irregular Heartbeats

Far too many reputable cardiologists are stating that their many years as practitioners in this field of specialty have shown that these irregular heartbeats are very common and very rarely pose a health threat to otherwise healthy people (some cardiologists even call them "normal"). They add statements to this fact, saying to the effect that PVCs/PACs rarely have any diagnostic significance and many of these doctors admit to experiencing them their selves. Keep in mind that we are talking about irregular heartbeats, rather than chronic arrhythmias (an ongoing rather than intermittent change in cardiac rhythm).

Stress and Anxiety: Major Triggers for Palpitations

I also want to remind, that people, who anticipate PVCs/PACs, due to their fear of them, are actually contributing to more of them (certainly not their fault but a natural response). Also, when one occurs, it tends to cause a quick surge of adrenaline in the body, due to the anxiety these palpitations may cause (fight or flight response) and this will instantly trigger succeeding PVCs/PACs, possibly several of them in a row. For this reason, people who are under chronic stress or anxiety can experience them with more frequency than do people who have other triggers for them (i.e. caffeine, following exercise or lack of sleep).

Cardiologist - Dr. Michael G. Kienzle, MD says this regarding PVCs:

"...PVCs are common. In the vast majority of cases, they are of no prognostic significance and frequently go away on their own without any treatment beyond being reassured by your doctor."

While it is my hope that this chapter has also provided a bit of comfort to those who may be experiencing these skips and jumps in their heart rhythm, I do want to again remind that any type of heart arrhythmia should be further evaluated by a qualified doctor, as a wise precaution.

CHAPTER FOUR

Common Treatments for Heart Palpitations

(Lifestyle, Pharmaceutical and Natural Solutions for PVCs and PACS)

Magnesium and Potassium Supplementation

Studies of people with PVCs and PACs have revealed that they are often low in one or both of these essential minerals that have a great deal to do with healthy heart function. When these necessary elements in the body become low or are at sub-normal levels, this can contribute to arrhythmias such as tachycardia, skipped beats, flip-flops and flutters. Taking a safe supplementation-dose of magnesium and/or potassium as overseen by a medical professional, may help to control these symptoms and also contribute to overall better heart-health. To determine if a patient with palpitations is low in magnesium and/or potassium, a qualified doctor would first need to order mineral analysis tests, by blood or hair sample.

Beta-blocker Medications

Beta-adrenergic blocking agents or "beta-blockers" are medications that control blood pressure irregularities, especially hypertension (high blood pressure) which can also be a co-occurring symptom or even a cause of heart palpitations. It can also help to regulate blood pressure changes that patients with palpitations can experience with positional changes of their body or their "postural blood pressure".

In addition to this, the medication can help reduce spells of tachycardia and diminish the effects of anxiety and panic symptoms that are experienced, by blocking some of the effects of adrenaline that tends to be overactive in many patients with skipped heartbeats and rapid heart rate.

Avoid Stimulants

Patients who experience concerning palpitations need to reduce or completely eliminate the amount of stimulants in their diets. These would be things including alcohol, caffeine, and refined sugar (added sugar not occurring naturally in foods).

Elimination of these can help control symptoms of anxiety and arrhythmias and help to keep stress-levels down which can also contribute to symptoms.

Reduce Stress and Drink Water

Stress, in fact is also a stimulant that needs to be reduced as much as possible due to its effect in also contributing-to and aggravating heart palpitations. Patients with bothersome palpitations should also remain well-hydrated, meaning they should drink plenty of water which helps to keep blood volume at the correct level. If there is not adequate water intake, blood volume can drop, causing a condition called "hypovolemia", which can contribute to symptoms of fatigue, dizziness and heart rhythm disturbances.

The Benefits of Regular Exercise

Regular exercise at a safe pace and at a well-tolerated level can also reduce stress and help to keep the involuntary nervous system better balanced in regulating blood pressure and heart rhythm.

Are Common Heart Skip Palpitations Dangerous?

35

Exercise has also been found in research studies to help reduce anxiety and depression levels, as well as-do medications that are also designed for this. Should a patient with frequent PVCs or PACS also need the help of an anti-anxiety or antidepressant medication or emotional therapies these should also be considerations in helping them to cope with symptoms and to regain a better quality-of-life.

Types of anti-anxiety medications (benzodiazepines) include the following:

• alprazolam (Xanax®)

• clonazepam (Klonipin®)

• lorazepam (Ativan®)

• diazepam (Valium®)

• buspirone (Buspar®) (this one is a azaspirodecanedione class drug)

Types of anti-depressants (selective serotonin reuptake inhibitors) that also work as anti-anxiety medications include the following:

• paroxetine (Paxil®) ...

Are Common Heart Skip Palpitations Dangerous?

...

- venlafexine (Effexor®)

- fluoxetine (Prozac®)

- setraline (Zoloft®)

- fluvoxamine (Luvox ®)

In regard to psychiatric therapies, one that is highly successful in treating anxiety disorders and conditions of all kinds is "Cognitive Behavioral Therapy" (CBT). This method can be administered by a qualified mental health professional or in some cases; it can be self-administered via programs than can be used in the privacy of one's home. I do suggest however that home programs found by online search or at bookstores, have the endorsement or involvement of a psychiatric doctor or a reputable mental health association.

Get Complete Blood Tests

As previously mentioned, minerals such as magnesium and potassium can become low in the body.

Are Common Heart Skip Palpitations Dangerous?

These are also in the "electrolyte" category and several other nutrients are as well, including phosphate and sodium. Imbalances in these can affect heart function as well if they fall significantly outside of normal values -- whether levels become abnormally low or abnormally high in the body. Blood tests can also detect abnormal levels of vitamins (i.e. B12, D and B6) and hormone levels (i.e. sex, adrenal and thyroid hormones), all of which can also affect heart function when they become significantly imbalanced. Hyperthyroidism for example (overactive thyroid gland), can cause heart palpitations, such as sustained tachycardia and correction of the hormone imbalance can restore normal heart rhythm. These reasons are why it is important to ask one's doctor for complete blood tests, to detect potential causes of heart palpitations. This will allow-for treatment of such underlying causes that might be found, which can improve or even completely correct the occurrence of PVCs, PACs and other common heart arrhythmias.

Are Common Heart Skip Palpitations Dangerous?

In Conclusion:

These often concerning but common and treatable heart palpitations do not have to disrupt a person's life any more than necessary, when methods for identifying causes or contributing factors are used, followed by administration of best-possible treatments for them. In many cases, self-administered lifestyle changes can greatly assist in treatment, in addition to that which may be required under the supervision of a medical doctor. In-short, sufferers of frequent PVCs and PACs can be assured that they will recover quality-of-life by being proactive in their treatment.

I offer my sincerest "Best Wishes" to the readers of this section, who undertake such remedies for their benign but emotionally-impacting heart palpitations and I thank you for reading the information I have offered!

(END)